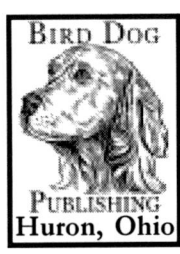

HEART MURMURS

POEMS

JOHN A. VANEK

To Don,
Wishing you love + long life
with no lament
   Jack Vanek

BIRD DOG PUBLISHING
HURON, OHIO

© 2009 Bird Dog Publishing
& John Vanek
ISBN 978-1-933964-27-0

Bird Dog Publishing
An Imprint of Bottom Dog Press
PO Box 425
Huron, Ohio 44839
http://smithdocs.net
e-mail Lsmithdog@smithdocs.net

CREDITS:

Cover art by Matthew Vanek
Book & Cover design by Susanna Sharp-Schwacke
Author photo by William Stickley
General Editor: Larry Smith

ACKNOWLEDGMENTS:

We would like to thank the following publications in which these poems, some in earlier versions, first appeared or are scheduled to appear:

Small Brushes: "Permanent Record" and "Living Color"
Heartlands: "The People's Republic," "Orphaned at Fifty, I Pack Up My Childhood Bedroom and Find," "Waltzing with Roethke," "Those Left Behind," and "Good Friday at the Art Museum"
Pennsylvania Poetry Society Prize Poems 2005: "The Poem I Would Write" and "Valediction for Mikey"
Bloodroot Literary Review: "Double Feature," "There Are Days," and "Balloons"
Confluence: "The Changing Room"
Turtlequill Journal of the Literary Arts: "The Hardest Thing," "Always, Autumn Leaves," "Chest X-ray," and "In Another Time"
Ascent Aspirations Magazine - Wildfire Anthology (Canada): "Appetites"

(Continued on page 121.)

Contents

Foreword: On *Heart Murmurs* 9
Prologue: Permanent Record 11

I – Longing

The People's Republic 15
The Poem I Would Write 16
Double Feature 17
The Changing Room 18
The Hardest Thing 19
Always, Autumn Leaves 20
There Are Days 21
Appetites 22
Isthmus Pantoum 23
Monsters and Ghosts 24
Wonderland 25
Great Lake Gusts 26
Horizontal Tears 27
Orphaned at Fifty, I Pack Up My Childhood Bedroom and Find 28
A Miss America Pageant Finalist 29
Desire 30

II – Love

Bordeaux Simple 33
Piano Recital: Homage to Maurice Ravel 34
They 35
Ordinary Miracles 36
Squall 37
Mr. Fix-It 38
Mood Music 39
You and I 40
Constant 41
Waltzing with Roethke 42
I'm Six 43
Addiction Tanka 44
Anatomy of Love 45

III – Lament

Balloons 49
Another Found Poem 50
Black and White Photograph 52
Crosses Along the Highway 53
September Bloom 54

Portable Memories...55
Rocks..56
A Day Like Any Other...57
Manhattan Streets...58
Glass of Absinthe—Picasso 1911, Oil on Canvas........................59
Twenty-One Gun Tanka...61
Shrapnel..62
Extra Innings...63
Chest X-ray..65
Bedside...66
Valediction for Mikey...67
The Unbearable Weight of Ashes..68
Those Left Behind..69
Chains...70
Pediatric Oncology..71
The God of Broken Things..72
Good Friday at the Art Museum...74

IV – LIFE

Living Color...77
Sea Shell...78
Brown Anole..79
Between..80
Rice Paper Seasons..81
Blackbird..82
In Another Time...84
Positive...85
The Tough Trek Home...86
Hindsight..87
Silence..88
Matthew 5:49...89
Finding the Words..90
Essence...91
Generic Novel..92
My Muse...93
Ode to Glory..94
Reservations...95
The World's Sexiest Man..97
Marilyn, What Is It Like...98
Jesus Left Me Today...99
Snapshots at a Wedding...100
Seasoned Citizens: Thirteen Ways of Looking at Gray Birds....101
Worship..104
Ageless..105

Feeling Invisible 106
Hangin' with Grandma 107
Downhill 108
Sepia World 110
Oberlin 112
Georgia O'Keeffe—A Found Poem 114
When I Dreamt of Daughters 116
Grail 118

Foreword: On *Heart Murmurs*

I am a physician by training and a poet by passion. I discovered the healing properties of poems as I dealt with my mother's Alzheimer's disease, my father's death from cancer, the suicide of a family friend, and the suffering I witnessed in my medical practice. Poetry provided a vehicle that took me to places that logic wouldn't go. It became a way of understanding the incomprehensible, both in life and in medicine. I now prescribe poetry PRN ("as needed"), but warn that "it may hurt a little."

Although this book is a work of fiction, any resemblance to actual events or persons is not entirely coincidental. My poetry is peopled with friends, family, and patients who live in the heartland and in my heart.

Dedication

For Geni, Matt, and Jess,
whose murmurs are always in my heart,
and for the fine poets who guided me on this journey.

Permanent Record

My children discover my childhood
locked up like a bird in a shoebox.
They toss the top off and out flies Miss Black,
our second grade teacher, my report card clutched
in a claw-full of knuckles:

Johnny grapples with grammar,
labors with language,
struggles with sounds,
rambles when writing.
Let's hope he persists.

Now forty years later, every syllable flows
quite slowly still from my tongue
and my pen, each word thick
and sweet
as savored honey.

Longing

And the day came when the risk it took to remain tight inside the bud was more painful than the risk it took to blossom.
— Anais Nin

The People's Republic

A communist, half a world away
from his terra-cotta life in Xian,
Lai never actually said
he loved America;
he just savored her
like a concubine.

From my deck we watched
an arrowhead of geese
pierce a cloud,
as sunset melted over the marshland
and warm breezes launched lake ripples
like a comb through hair.

Total-body baptized in the Church
of Capitalism, Lai looked up
from his New Testament,
Consumer Reports,
to watch swallows
swirl like a waterspout across the bay—

then he returned to a gospel so foreign
it seemed written by a higher power.
He said he had faith that someday
his government would grant him a refrigerator…
but stumbled mid-sentence
as the distant *crack* of a rifle

emptied the marsh,
and saturated the sky
with birds proclaiming
their inalienable rights.
He recoiled, then sighed,
as a hundred sorrows floated

in his half moon eyes.
He said that in his province
there were no birds.
His angular features wilted,
and from a place of silk and sadness, he added,
"We ate them all."

The Poem I Would Write

If I wasn't so tired, I would compose
a symphony of sounds,
unleashing the evening's dark desires
as a tympani of consonants
drumming the hair on your neck to attention

and before you knew what was happening,
march you quick-time to the second stanza,
where I'd introduce the melody,
disguised as the whisper of a silk dress
dancing between long legs,

then counterpoint with the music
of a nightingale,
sliding into a minor key
to make you weep, each word
an echo of your longing, and I'd

watch you sigh between stanzas,
breathe between lines, seducing you
with subtle harmonies of rhyme, flutes
of champagne,
the moon's satin shoulders, until

the staccato of high heels across marble,
of full lips untouching,
create a crescendo of urgency,
and you begin to see
what we all know

engulfed in the darkness, not of the nightingale,
but the little black dress
fluttering to the floor in the final stanza,
having served its purpose,
at rest at last.

Double Feature

You live life like a car chase, your sweat
just spent rubber on the office floor,
as you fly in a vintage blue convertible
desperately searching for something,
anything, like Thelma and Louise,
always looking over your shoulder
for cops in the rearview, as if
you just robbed a liquor store
or shot someone for no good reason,
no time to think, to reflect,
just react, stand on the gas pedal
trying not to spin out, flip over,
flip out, knowing the ending
will be funny, tragically funny,
when suddenly tires screech
as you arrive at the edge
of the Grand Canyon, and they
present you with a handshake
and a gold watch that melts,
runs through your arthritic fingers
like a Dali painting, while you
peer over the cliff

and you are in an Ingmar Bergman film.
Life is black and white and slow.
You sit at a table, conversing
in Swedish, a language
you do not understand.
You stroll with a striking, young thing,
lusting after god-knows-what.
You ride with your son in a Studebaker, drowning
as the car fills with indifference.
Then, you are at your desk,
writing your autobiography,
but completely lose interest.
You begin to wonder how you lived life without
knocking off a liquor store,
and you wonder about the accelerator,
the cliff,
and whether you could make it
to the other side of the canyon.

The Changing Room

Like picking men, she thinks,
as she grabs another gown
with festive hospital logos.
Never know where they've been.

She tries not to knot her hair
tying bows behind her back,
then dances with the mirror,
her reflection *elegant yet sassy*

in a bile-green gown.
She leaves her socks on
as if embarrassed by naked feet;
squirrels her clothes in a hookless locker

with the keys and the smile
she hangs every night by the door;
shudders at the rush of cold air
from the bottom, the back,

the sleeves her arms no longer fill;
shudders at her transformation
as she waits for her name to be called,
waits while cells divide; then

gazes at the radiation tattoo
on her breast,
before emerging
from the changing room.

The Hardest Thing: A Voice

How strange to hear my thoughts echo,
ricochet inside my mind, unable to exit
my muted mouth, the hinges rusted shut.
For eighty years, ideas departed this gray station
like train cars, each coupled to the next,
every sentence latched to another.
Now, one bell short of midnight forever,
I can't even curse
or shake my fist at God.

My grandchild plants wild flowers
in a cup on the nightstand, a kiss on my cheek.
The fool's gold of December
pours between clouds like a Bible painting, lighting
her pumpkin hair, a child-face.
She quenches my thirst
with ice chips, lemon sticks,
tales of volleyball, dances,
a boy. I have no words.

Why did I wait until my stricken tongue
was stuck between my teeth
to tell her to *live life*
not as a noun, but as a verb:
to explore, experience, emerge,
contemplate, challenge, conquer,
sample, sin, savor,
laugh, lament, love.
All that I never told her, I can't tell her now.

She hugs my half-lifeless body,
watches me lift my right hand
with my left.
I don't know how to comfort this girl
who wipes drool from my mouth,
tears from adolescent eyes
crying out to change what can't be.
And though clinging to life with only one hand
makes letting go easier, for me

the hardest thing
is not being
the saddest in the room.

ALWAYS, AUTUMN LEAVES
a villanelle

It is strange how life clings to the last:
The red one is stoic, knows the way of the seasons,
yet looks warily down at green grass.

The brown one is wrinkled and lives in the past,
considers deserting the family as treason.
It is strange how life clings to the last.

The yellow remembers all those who have passed,
views the end as mere fate, not logic or reason,
so lies willingly down in the grass.

The dark one flies like a flag on a mast,
more purple than black, in sunset's last crimson—
it is strange how some cling to the last.

From my hospital window, fall's colors bleed fast,
for this tubing's my stem, both lifeline and prison,
as I wait for parole to green grass.

This evening, I'm fragile and pale as veined glass,
yet reach out for my lover, our daughter, her son.
It is strange how I cling to the last,
yet look longingly down at green grass.

There Are Days

In the painting on my easel, a woman
leans against a gate at twilight, her eyes
dead as the graveyard beneath her, her frame so slight
the weight of a smile, anyone's smile,
might crush her.

Her pursed lips sing a dirge without words.
A rag doll hangs limp from one hand, the other
holds her heart in her chest, as Venetian red
seems to bleed through the canvas
of her blouse.

Time blows like a breeze
through her veil
of gray hair, the light wind
a gentle hand
of sympathy on her shoulder.

Maybe I should paint her eyes closed,
arms open, as if sleepwalking
in a dream of ambulance lights,
as if she feels the phantom kick
of an empty womb,

as if she knows
that everyone's final breath
waits somewhere deep inside.
Maybe I should paint my own eyes
closed to suffering.

The sky is black wallpaper;
the air is silver smoke.
You may see it differently, but I suspect
she has already cast her hope
in the bonfire of good intentions.

I wish she would leave
the painting, my studio,
turn her gaze from me.
There are days I wish
I could lay down my brush.

APPETITES

Protected only by animal skin,
we whirl through dusky perfumes,
hearts thumping ancient rhythms.
Our senses drone louder than insects,
hum a dark tune—prelude
to our own inevitable duet.

    Her long legs
    tango with the night,
    lure ravenous eyes
    like crazed fireflies.

    Savoring, he circles,
    invisible as longing,
    muscle fibers flickering
    beneath taut skin, then

        he thrusts   his great weight upon her   collapses
her card-table legs   as she   lashes back   their eyes
    clenched like wrestlers   both alive in the bite
of teeth and nails   both craving climax   'til the heat
    of the rending   sets them ablaze.

    Need incarnate, beasts
    without claws, we tremble—
    as the sweet, open-market scent
    of fresh flesh
    brings our own blood-soup
    to a tantalizing boil.

Isthmus Pantoum

The two of us stand,
both trembling with fear,
on Love's isthmus of sand,
as cross-currents rush near.

We're living in fear
for we each hold Love's knife.
Is that storm growing near
just the roar of our strife?

Love's double-edged knife
poised to whittle two trees
on our isthmus of strife,
trust tossed in the breeze.

Two frail wind-whipped trees
and a few grains of sand—
a staunch nor'east breeze
and two islands stand.

Monsters and Ghosts

We play a round of *Patty Cake*,
her fingers dwarfed by mine.
Cat's Cradle erupts in claps of joy,
surprise in her smile.

Together we search for monsters
in closets and under the bed—'til night
waltzes circles around us, dances me back
to my internship:

> to a child of a woman, face
> eclipsed by draped knees,
> ebony skin, pink through the speculum,
> scarlet in the surgical basin.

> My mentor whispers: *Hold the curette*
> *like an artist's brush, the razor bristles*
> *slicing down to muscle.*   Scrape.
> *Feel the grating resistance.*   Scrape.

> Then a tiny hand emerges, nails painted
> with blood, fingers clutching
> the teeth of the cold curette, and I learn
> how some stains never wash clean.

Tender palms cradle my stubble,
tremble like the voice in my ear:
Daddy! Daddy! I can't sleep.
Our fears are left unsaid—

muted by moans in the closet,
monsters shuffling under the bed.

Wonderland

Growing up is never quite fair
        to babies—or parents whose lives they disrupt.
Let's hope that God hears small prayers.

Our toddlers engender both joy and despair—
        kid soldiers court-martialed for disorderly conduct.
Growing up has never been fair.

Soon the house overflows with stuffed tigers and bears,
        toy trains, board games, boyfriends, and makeup.
And let's hope some god hears our prayers

when our teens seize the world as if it were theirs.
        Love builds up; they break up; we mop up.
Growing older is often unfair.

The Mad Hatter's watch makes us finally aware
        how days whirl by when the little hand speeds up.
Let's hope that God hears our prayers.

Though arthritic hands deal our last solitaire,
        the game's end can be either prolonged or abrupt.
Growing old is never quite fair.
Let's hope that God hears all prayers.

Great Lake Gusts

When the blast furnace fire
flickered and died, Papa retired
his last paycheck
at the *Iron Bar and Grill*,
garaged his steel-toed shoes,
shuffled once-white socks
across kitchen linoleum
past the Formica breakfast nook
into the breezeway.

Casting his great weight
into the rocking chair, he
hardened like metal in a mold,
his sausage legs
lumpy and cracked as the skin
of his hassock, the neck
of his beer bottle
like an extra thumb
on his catcher's-mitt-sized hand.

He synchronized his sway
with the whistle of each wheeze
and the flap of yellow laundry
in the industrial breeze, until
he closed his eyes
that final time.

I thought I saw him this morning
on the porch at *Cracker Barrel*,
by the potbellied stove
with no fire in its belly,
sitting with Elmer, his identical twin,
strangled at seven by whooping cough—
thought I heard his creak
among the cane-backed rockers
nodding with each Great Lake gust,
each heartland breath.

HORIZONTAL TEARS
for Dad

......and into the windowless room with blinking slot machines
and fluorescent hum he walks, and I recognize the thin gray hair,
a hint of Aqua Velva, that faded madras shirt he always wore, though
I haven't seen it in years, and I remember he always loved Vegas,
blackjack, the glitz, and when we embrace, Dad feels so warm,
so wonderfully warm I can't let go, though he keeps shuffling
forward as I keep sliding back, and I ask how he is and he
says *Okay,* but doesn't smile, doesn't look at me, and I
realize how much I miss him, so I hang on, though
Dad is almost out of the room, and I know it's
not possible, but tears are streaming from my
left eye, horizontally across my nose, so
it's no surprise the pillow is soaked,
for he's been gone three years,
and I know it will be forever
before this shaking stops,
longer before I can sleep,
dream again, as I lie here
waiting for his return,
knowing I may never
hold him again......

Orphaned at Fifty, I Pack Up My Childhood Bedroom and Find

I am the sum of inconsequential things:
trophies of golden plastic, teen treasures,
remnants of tears and triumphs
enshrined by my mother
in this mausoleum of my youth.

I am the bow, hardwood
pulled taut by frayed string,
grooved by the flight of errant arrows
launched by a crazed Cupid, always piercing
the heart of the wrong lover.

I am the Swiss army knife,
a white cross on a field of blood
shed in the heat of an Asian war,
my tempered steel blade
dulled, collapsed inward.

I am the river stone, polished smooth
against others of my kind
in icy Ohio streams,
the imprint of ancestors
fossilized in the hard grit within.

A Miss America Pageant Finalist

    in her mind, dressed to the "nines"
in a binary world on a nude beach,
    she wades ankle-deep and wonders

whether to come out of the water
    or sound its depths, yet
hypnotized by the horizon

    she waits for a ship
that will never come in,
    waits for the hand of God,

or any hand,
    to transport her
to some Shangri-La by the sea.

Desire

is alive, a growing thing.
Unattended, it drifts
like a mushroom spore
on winds of capricious thought
to the dank loam in a shady nook
of the mind, where
it suckles the damp marrow

of sweat, solitude, selfishness—
burgeoning into full-bodied
succulent lust—
dangerous as the ivory-capped
Destroying Angel,
Amanita virosa,[1]
deadly as original sin, yet

if nurtured in warmth and sunlight,
it can flower like genus *Odontoglossum,*[2]
each touch of tongue,
tender nibble of teeth,
budding into floral fantasy,
blossoming into the passion
of an *Angel Star Orchid.*

---

[1] The *Amanita* group of mushrooms contains amanitin, one of the deadliest poisons found in nature. One cap of a *Destroying Angel* can kill.

[2] *Odontoglossum,* from the Greek words *odon* (tooth) and *glossa* (tongue), is a genus of 100 orchids, of which *Angel Stars* are among the most elegant.

LOVE

Fragrance always clings to the hand that gives the rose.
—Chinese proverb

Bordeaux Simple

On a hillside, on a blanket,
on our third glass of red,
as I listen to her hair
whisper on bare shoulders, she
leans into mocha dusk and asks:
*What first attracts you
to a woman?*

And there is no escape. Curves
sashay through my mind as night
binds me like a straitjacket.
I want to say the answer
is more like Burgundy than Bordeaux,
complicated, though it's not.
I think I might tell her the "eyes"
but can't see hers in the darkness
and haven't yet learned their color.

She carefully breaks the bread
and my silence, my body
stuttering, as I flick away
crumbs like doubts. Then a truth
I never knew existed
tumbles from my lips:
The smile, I say.
*Not the window to the soul, but
the gateway.*

And in that moment, life
is Bordeaux simple,
as Burgundy lips part,
the door swings open
bright and white,
and she welcomes me in.

Piano Recital: Homage to Maurice Ravel

The up and down and up and down again
of knuckled hammers striking ebony,
while ivory pistons pound their felt on wire
both up and down and up and down until
like bows on violins and padded sticks
on tympani an orchestra appears
conducted by Ravel himself, each rise
and fall of striking strings like stormy waves
upon the fleshy drums inside my head.

Through closing eyes I see a flowered dress
cavorting with the wildflowers as
all blossoms merge into a meadow scene,
her graceful footfalls in the subtle bass
are softened by piano pedal's touch,
and I can only chase her memory,
await her second coming into view,
anticipate the murmur of her clothes,
her laughter in the treble song of birds—

the sum: a growing rumble at my core
that sweeps us toward the torrent's waterfall,
the last arpeggio demands we soar
beyond the edge and gliding fall at last
back to the room where fingers up and down
embrace the final notes—as I caress
the alabaster hand of joy and gaze
upon the dappled dress that blossoms on
the girl who smiles and nods, her eyes still closed.

THEY

She is the freckled evening sky,
He, the shooting star, their nights
      dazzling meteor showers.

He is the swirl of the storm,
She, the calm eye, dancing
      in step with his lead.

She is the doe in dawn stillness,
He, the owl, restless eyes
      searching the night.

He is the river's current,
She, bedrock,
      his foundation.

She is the acorn nestled in loam,
He, the maple seed
      whirling over rocky soil.

He is the wild strawberry in the briar patch,
She, the ripened peach
      reaching toward outstretched hands.

She is the frost-kissed fir,
He, the fire-bush burning
      red on the grass.

He is the match at the kindling,
She, cupped hands in the wind,
      both warmed.

She is the winter wheat,
He, the scythe—together
      they are the harvest.

Ordinary Miracles

Love is easy as herding
    hummingbirds, a simple gathering
of morning mist.

From opposite banks they wade
    into water
sweetened by her reflection.

He pans for gold flecks
    in fluid blue eyes,
his face

lit up by fiery hair
    that flows through his fingers
like laughter,

as gentle currents
    gather them toward
their moment.

She listens to his heart,
    to sounds
she's never heard,

her face a perfect fit
    between his chest and cheek,
his smile

an extension of hers. Together, they are
    a two-piece jigsaw puzzle
completed.

So when he asks,
    she agrees, and God
embraces another

ordinary miracle,
    hummingbirds on His shoulders,
pockets filled with morning mist.

SQUALL

You sense sharp edges
in the air, the aroma
of rot and renewal, a chill
in the restive wind, yet

this summer rainstorm is all bluster.
Silence explodes, not in thunder, but the popping
of plump raindrops, like ripe tomatoes
smacking pavement

with the sting of hurled insults,
the drops so far apart
the memory lingers on the sidewalk
in a mosaic of wet and dry.

Then, with a distant flash,
a low rumble
more groan than growl,
it's gone—

like anger
after a spat
over nothing important,
the concrete already drying.

Mr. Fix-It

One little Swiss couple
has stumbled from the dance hall, so I
glue them on their pedestal
to the cheers of the cuckoo, then

rehab the delinquent towel rack
that slouches like James Dean,
shrugging off facecloths,
a pair of her stockings.

The alarm clock blinks *12:00*, yet time
is but a concept, sleep a nightmare.
And why bother to attach the white king's head,
gazing from the board at the dark queen's feet?

Though, I must repair the red clay ashtray
our daughter made,
missile-launched by her mother
in our latest battle—another casualty of war.

It's strange that I know how to fix leaking faucets,
yet have no idea how to stop the trickle
from my eyes, or what to do with these ten nails,
bloodied, gnawed to the quick.

Mood Music

A barstool clairvoyant
alone on the deck, hair combed back
by a petulant gale,
I look upon a storm-stirred sea

rabid with foam, flotsam
tossed like tea leaves,
and try to divine
our future.

I tilt my long neck
Molson Golden
so the wind's weathered lips
blow a somber sound

across its cold glass mouth,
each note lower
than the sip before, falling
with my mood.

You and I

You once told me: "There is no *I* in *love*"—
though with us, I've learned
there's often a *lo*.

I was in every *kiss*,
and it's no surprise
there is an *us* in *lust*.

For me, there's always been a *yes*
in the sparkle of your *eyes*, a definite *high*
in the touch of your *thigh*.

Elation beat at the heart of our *relationship*, yet
I feared that if we got too *close*,
I could only *lose*.

If only I hadn't panicked when you said
we were destined to *wed*, though *if* is the point
around which *life* pivots.

Engagements just seems to *age men*, so
when we became a *couple*, all I could see
was a *coup*, the violent overthrow of me.

I guess *I* embody *insensitivity*, yet it's ironic
that when you had an *affair*, it was only *fair*,
but when I took a *lover*, we were *over*.

Now you say: "We can still be *friends?*"—
which everyone knows
is how happiness *ends*.

And though there will never be an *I* in *love*,
you should know, as you walk out the door,
that I will never

not be in love with you.

Constant

Today, in the attic,
I unearth this outdated globe
with country names and boundaries
all wrong,

then discover the mobile
that circled my son's crib,
watch planets whirl
to *You Are My Sunshine*.

So I phone my boy, but his mother
says he's not home—
and the vacuum of space
in my bed

sucks me under the covers,
where I read in the paper
that fact is fluid,
truth transient, read

that for twenty years
Neptune and Pluto switched places
like gods in a footrace,
with Neptune trailing strides behind.

Yet, as fast as I sprint
I go nowhere,
will never even catch Saturn,
whose rings

are the shape of love
abandoned, the pallid shape
of untanned skin
circling my finger,

constant as stardust,
as *I'll love you forever*.

Waltzing with Roethke

I read your poems and cry out,
for I was never blessed
with a papa who caressed me

with buckles, who held his whiskey
with the same battered knuckles
that beat me, never blessed

with a mother whose hands preferred
the touch of cast iron and copper
to my embrace.

    I wonder how you sired
    beautiful poems, like children,
    strong and unblemished,

    how you buried old scars
    close enough to your skin
    to be felt yet not seen,

    how you built your life
    stretched taut on the framework
    of those fibrous struts.

        A geyser explodes
        from the bottomless spring
        of my son's brush onto canvas.

        I smile a father's smile
        but wonder why the reds
        are so bloody, the blacks so bleak,

        wonder where he found a palette
        with colors that cut, hues that hurt—
        then shaking, take my waking slow.

I'm Six

but use all sixty-four crayons
to draw a house that looks
like a smiling face:
bright-eyed windows,
ruby-lipped door,
a rainbow necklace of flowers—
and I always,
always color
inside the lines, because
that usually
makes them happy.

Addiction Tanka

My last drag is so
long and deep, the tip glows red
as an angry eye,
the smoke sears hot and hurtful
like a love that never quits.

ANATOMY OF LOVE

When I say I "love" you, I mean
the moonlight dancing across your hair
reflects from the mirror that is you
in splendid full light spectrum,
and your rainbow beauty is focused
by lenses onto my retinas, then carried like a bride
across the threshold of the optic nerves,
overloading my neural network
like faulty wiring
on a brittle-brown Christmas tree,
and from the top branch, I hear
the pineal gland murmur: "The night is young!"
as my olfactory lobes detect the smell of smoke,
and hormones spray
from a pituitary sprinkler
filling my blood with adrenaline jet fuel,
causing my diaphragms to pump like bellows,
sucking a tornado of night air down my trachea,
stars and all, lifting me like a helium balloon,
as my pulsing aorta takes all the flow
the old ticker can muster, temporal arteries
beating my head like twin tom-toms until
I whirl in a vertigo dance, the rush of red cells
flooding my cheeks, ears, and loins
causing both chambers of my corpus cavernosum
to engorge, and well, you know…
yet I barely can hear my appendix
drone endlessly on
about feeling neglected, useless,
because the auditory nerves are ringing
church bells in my ears, as every cell
lights up like the 4th of July,
and combustible emotions
ignite in the hippocampus and amygdala,
burn across the medulla, down my spinal cord like a fuse,
sodium and calcium ion channels opening
as muscles contract, my lips part,
and I take you in my arms for a deep kiss—so,
don't you smirk and roll your eyes and tell me
I don't know the meaning of "love,"
'cause baby, I'm up to my anus in degrees,
and I *wrote* the damn textbook
on *love*!

Lament

*Heavy hearts, like heavy clouds, are best relieved
by the letting of a little water.*
—Christopher Morley

BALLOONS
for Joel

My son's best friend, six years
in remission,
leaves the pre-prom party, comes to me,
puts a hand on my shoulder,
sits, says I look sad.

I tell him, *I'm fine*,
cloak my deceit
in a throaty laugh,
ask why he's not
inside flirting.

Joel just shrugs, as if he has
a lifetime of time, says
he's spreading his wings, soaring
to Florida this fall for college.
His smile warms the cold Ohio spring,

refills my deflating middle age
with the lightness of possibility.
Then he's gone—
back to the party, worrying about
finals, graduation, prom night.

Three years later, his friends
gather in an early April drizzle, each
clinging to the string of a helium balloon.
Mine is red, my son's is green,
Joel's Mom's is blue.

When the eulogy ends, we let them go,
bleeding all color from Ohio
into a polka dot sky.
I guess I'll always see
those damn balloons

and his smile in my mind until
the sky dons a polka dot rainbow
for me.
I hug my son, afraid to let go,
afraid he'll float away.

Another Found Poem

Christmas lights of red and green
twinkle on the monitor,
flash pulse and pressure, proclaim
the baby in this crib will live
for now.

My gloved hand hovers above the only vein
on his hairless scalp, 'til the butterfly
needle finds courage to land,
and I tape the tube to sallow skin
that wants to tear away.

Blue fingers fist with the whoosh
of each breath, as bellows fan
this fading ember—a warm blanket
and a mother's sleepless song,
gifts for the newborn child.

She huddles with her husband as if cold,
his blue blazer now her shawl, limbs and lives
entwined, nestled forehead to forehead,
exchanging a dialysis
of toxic hope.

I want nothing more
than the sleep of a silent night
filled with dreams of places
other than here, heedless
of her cradlesong.

In this strawless manger of sorrow,
below a fluorescent star, I wonder
how to tell this couple
the baby they never could bear
will be gone by New Year's.

I fiddle with knobs, gauge
how much they understand,
snatch glances meant for each other,
stare at my blood-spattered shoes, then
tell them—

and all is lost
but these words
and the haunting hum
of a mother's
never-ending lullaby.

Black and White Photograph

Maybe the gallery on Fifth Street
is possessed, but you can't walk past.
Lured inside the photo of a motel room,
you stumble over black boots by the nightstand,
wipe dust from an unopened Bible.

Next to a half bottle of Southern Comfort,
a jackknife impales both the desk
and front page snapshot of a man
who bleeds on a balcony,
the headline reading, "King Killed!"

The windup clock marks time.
The radio dial glowers. You can almost
hear the news.
And on the door hook hang
a motorcycle jacket and leather pants,

like the skin of a black man
deep in an Alabama woods.

Crosses Along the Highway

On a stretch of I-75 between Lexington
and Knoxville, columns of crosses
flank the road's soft shoulders.

Some are wooden, paint chipping,
others stenciled with names, a few
sport baseball caps or

garlands of plastic flowers, and one
of lashed metal pipes
bleeds rust.

Another of celestial white soars
fifty feet into the heavenly blue, and I wonder
if this is the final resting place

of Paul Bunyan, clothes-lined by high tension wires
while chasing *Babe*, his ox.
Yet, bred and fed in the Bible Belt,

this cross ascends amid a gritty Gomorrah
and cinderblock Sodom, wedged
between Weapons World and the Porn Palace,

and I suspect that Jesus
suffocated here, the air
thick with despair.

September Bloom

The canoe slices dream-thick fog
toward curious blood red flowers
blooming among the lily pads
in absolute stillness.

Camouflaged amid
autumn's flotilla of leaves,
black eyes stare
from an iridescent green head,

wings edged in darkness,
chestnut breast and slate body
speckled scarlet, bloodied—a mallard,
capsized, scuttled, still.

Pluck a blood red flower,
half filled with water,
and the plastic petals read:
Bismuth Cartridge Company.

Feel the weight
of the brass base
with its single strike mark
and bold imprint: *twelve gauge*.

Portable Memories

Caught in a perilous place,
trapped in the flow of time,
the small dark life
that once was
silently buzzes in solid sunlight—
entombed in amber,
golden in my palm—
a portable memory.

I called her *Hoa Nho*,
Little Flower,
the only bloom in my world.
Her golden skin
was solid sunlight,
her hair an ebony veil,
dense and warm
as a jungle night.

For a dollar a week
she scrubbed the stench
of killing from my clothes.
I fed her rations
meant for our dead, fed her
Main Street dreams
like grapes and honey,
until she slept,

slept while the sticky
flow of time
trapped her wingless
in the napalm sap of 'Nam.

Rocks

Frogs complain like rusted hinges,
as swallows zigzag through cotton-candy fog
beneath a sleeping god's eyelids.
A Blue Heron sentry
protects his palace of riprap rock.

Head askew, he eyes the swallows
like a bachelor watching children
frolic on his crewcut lawn,
then scatters them
with a chain-smoker's rasp.

His White Heron neighbor to the north
takes three steps south. Pauses.
More steps. Waits. Stalemate.
Whitey advances and Old Blue
unfurls 747-sized wings,

launches low over the water
in slow-motion attack.
Whitey relocates closer to Canada,
as map makers
redraw the world atlas.

What is there about the homeland,
mein Heron? Why risk all
for that gnarled cluster of rock and weed,
those precious stones and sand
on which you make your stand?

Or Palestine? Tibet? Kashmir?
Israel? Or America?

A Day Like Any Other

Three miles apart, two girls comb their hair
just like any day, peer in the mirror, imagine
a world other than here, while strand by strand
the twine that ties hope to life unravels.

Tova paints pimples with a touch too much makeup,
prays for success in exams, for friends at the front,
shares a breakfast of challah
and chitchat with mother.

No manna for breakfast, Aya feasts
on the silence of loudspeakers
drained of broken Arabic, dines
on the absence of tanks, the curfew's end.

Given veils and trinkets when all she wants
is a weapon, Aya prays for dead brothers,
for success in her test, kisses her mother
goodbye, embraces her dowry of despair, then

stumbles through rubble for schooling
in manslaughter, and the Martyrs Brigade
stockpiles one more child-bomb in its arsenal,
videotapes her so the world will know

why the girl who dreamed of being a doctor,
when she still could dream, dispenses a dose
of suffering in the deli, swaddled in explosives
next to Tova.

Three miles apart, two mothers' tears
etch their flesh; a child's soft brown eyes
glaze and harden; men fire bullets and curses
skyward at someone's god.

While at the Wailing Wall
and the Dome of the Rock,
the stones remain silent,
just like any day.

Manhattan Streets

That corrosive flash of gas and glass
etched our retinas, denuded our optic nerves,
as gravity dragged us back to earth
and trust erupted into smoke and dust.

Shock-stilled, our dulled eyes darkened, while you
danced a demonic dance, robed in a guise of godliness,
showering your children with candy
in familial celebration of this demented holy day.

Soon, on a night when the sentry-moon is AWOL,
when only blindfolded Lady Justice
and the sightless can see,
you will dance no more—

then *we* shall weep for *all* children
as we hobble through the rubble,
guided only by our cane's returning echo
and our resolve.

When thermal burns finally heal and bandages unfurl,
we shall be colorblind with tunnel vision,
recognizing only those
who helped us safely cross

Manhattan streets.

GLASS OF ABSINTHE—PICASSO 1911, OIL ON CANVAS
Cocktails with Pablo, September 12, 2001

Tongue tinted bile green with absinthe,
you said: *Painting is the sum*
of destructions,
                    then
blew your beloved Paris Café
to life everlasting
on canvas—
                    now
a scrapheap of rust-etched metal,
jumbled stone shards,
decoupaged in a smoke blue hue.

At the top, fireplace remnants
flame, the exit blocked by debris.
Charred crates cube the cobbles
under fractured pillars, a severed staircase.

At the bottom, Napoleon's rakish hat
crowns a toppled chair
where no doubt you discussed
artful annihilation.

In this light, it's strange
        how the bronze bowl
        looks like a yarmulke,
        broken eyeglasses
        gaze from toppled towers,
        rust seems to ooze—

strange
        how this cone
        resembles the nose
        of an airship
        whose axle and wheels
        tumble to earth.

How much absinthe had you drunk, Pablo,
when you peered in that shattered mirror
and witnessed our world
plunge from the sky
yesterday?

---

* Picasso's painting, *Glass of Absinthe*, is on display at the Allen Memorial Art Museum in Oberlin, Ohio and can be viewed at http://www.oberlin.edu/amam/Picasso_Glass.htm

Twenty-One Gun Tanka

Seven set their sights
on Heaven; each fires three rounds
of blanks at God's eye,
brass jackets arcing to earth
like His electrified tears.

Shrapnel

Ice entombed leaves on the walk
shatter like childhood dreams.
I ease open the door
and await detonation.

She materializes, red rage rising
like mercury. Wrinkled hands
become fists. Frantic eyes
spark panic; her scowl smolders.

Tail a blur, old bones rattling like maracas,
my canine bomb squad licks
Mom's hand, captivating both
in a mariachi duet—

and hell fire is snuffed,
like spit-wet fingers on a match.

The rasp of a lock scrapes metal on metal,
beleaguered eyes peering
from a bathroom prison. My frail father
sighs as if pardoned by the governor.

I say that Mom's dementia is crushing him,
the burden's too great, that love
can't protect him, but my words
glance off old world ways.

I see the flame
re-ignite in her eyes before
the fuse hisses in my ear:
"Who are you?"

and my life is erased
by a simple question. Ka-boom.
Dad advances, tries to shield me,
arrives an instant too late.

Extra Innings

In sync with the TV,
youth flickers in cratered eyes
below a faded baseball cap
too large for its owner.

Baseball is like life, Dad whispers.
Tantalizes and torments, I reply.

Their center fielder
reaches over the fence,
pockets a homerun,
our joy in his glove.

It don't look good, he adds.
I don't disagree.

Stitched into our childhood,
our lives are measured in seasons
that stretch from early spring
well into fall, if the gods smile.

We circle the years like bases,
mesmerized by this game
with no time clock,
never knowing when it will end.

He naps between innings,
night between days,
then peers through mist
from his oxygen mask.

The vendor brings another round
of medicine, as rain
drips in his IV.
I steal moments, remembering

hope springs eternal,
but not forever.

We are bilingual,
but these days
speak only baseball,
for it is a language

without adjectives
like malignant or intractable,
or verbs like resuscitate, or nouns
like terminal.

We speak of relief
pitchers and pinch hitters,
try not to think about
the end of this season,

wait for a ninth inning miracle
to send him to extra innings
that we both know
will never come.

Chest X-ray

Bloated and globular, like Humpty Dumpty
sitting on a diaphragm wall, the heart
leans against the ribs,
as if sipping from a flask
waiting for the last train, dying
to bum a smoke.

If you listen, you can almost hear the lub-dub,
not of the train, but his syncopated song.
Nearby, parallel tracks glisten
calcium-white in the walls
of coronary arteries,
too brittle to carry the load.

If you gaze at the distant white-capped
apex of the lung, you'll see
the Dalai Lama, the all-knowing
cancer, holding the answers
to chaos, fingers
wrapped around the jugular.

And in the night-sky darkness
of the lungs, where hope diffuses,
pale scars and white-hot stars
of metastases
explode in a meteor shower
of a thousand possibilities

lost.

Bedside

You lie in utter stillness, so wasted
your robe appears uninhabited.
The angry hiss of oxygen
snakes through tubing,
and the scent of suffering
lingers in the night air.

Your remaining red cells effervesce,
carbonation from a spirit gone flat,
leaving you camouflaged in paleness
against a jungle of hospital sheets.
Skin so thin I fear
my touch will tear you.

Yet, you conjure up an impish grin,
as if you have a parting joke to tell—
while your eyes plead
for one last medical miracle
from a black bag that overflows
with hollow promises and jargon.

In the few gentle moments
when you sleep,
all I can do
is sit at your bedside,
write the elegy for your funeral,
and watch you wither.

Tonight, I will learn to live
a life without you—
if you
will find the faith
to close your eyes
one final time.

Valediction for Mikey

The note should have said:
Abandon hope, all who enter.
Instead it said: *Do not resuscitate*
my suffering.

His mind was a crown,
an austere and lonely garland
he wore for the world.
Thoughtful, he called his parents

the night before, strangely
to speak of nothing,
called in sick to work,
then washed dishes, paid bills

while waiting for neighbors to leave
for school or jobs.
He finished the twelve-page letter,
thankful for friendships,

grateful for family,
each name named, absolved—
the letter begun while waiting
the mandatory seven days

for the gunmetal blue light
Saturday night special.
He waited until
he could wait no longer,

until dying was as necessary
as breathing.
His mind was the crown
of thorns that pierced him bloody

for twenty-four years,
that solitary place
where he finally buried
the bullet.

The Unbearable Weight of Ashes
for Mikey

He recoiled from life
as abruptly as the echo
from the gunshot that took him,
leaving us staring
like severed heads on stakes
in the ringing silence.

Learning to live
with the decisions of the dead,
his parents share with us
aliquots of his ashes, as hallowed as hosts,
dispensed in tiny rosewood boxes
no one can shoulder.

Still, we make the obligatory appearances,
say the requisite good-byes,
and deliver our last full quota of tears—
until the wailing wind
scatters us
like hope and ashes.

Those Left Behind

Writhing on satin sheets, she
wrestles one worry too many
into the sunrise, a wilted rose
caged in a vase on the night stand.

On the table, a toppled bottle of Bordeaux
paints his portrait on the rug,
empty wine glasses count the days alone,
the reasons not to love.

She uncoils, awakes to a family
of shadows, expecting everything
but the dent in the mattress
where his body once lay,

the crater reminding those left behind
of the day the earth moved,
the climate changed, a hint of his cologne
hanging in the air like dust after impact.

Chains: A Voice

When I hear the jangle of chains,
the low growl, watch the fox
in the jaws of a trap
gnaw off her leg,

I taste blood again.

Our word is our bond,
Mao's little red book instructs,
yet collateral compels.
The Chairman knows which ties

bind like shackles, hobble bound feet.

For my student visa, he requires
my one-permitted child,
swaddled in the warm embrace
of the State, a red scarf

loosely knotted at her neck.

I take only a photo,
leave her in loyalty school
to learn comrade songs
I no longer can sing.

I leave the graves of my ancestors,

parents, dead spouse
and sail into an American sunset,
where streets are paved
with limitless children—

next time, maybe a boy.

Draped in stripes, in stars,
I sail my return ticket
from the bridge, then
cross the Golden Gate,

my stump barely visible.

Pediatric Oncology

There is no crystal staircase,
just a trek on tired feet
to the Fifth Floor, nearer to heaven,
as far as I can go.

This unfamiliar space is now
a shelter for my shifting life—this place
of misery, kindness, endings, beginnings—
where hugs are the currency of hope,

the cost of courage is sky-high,
and time's a fragile feast.
Where a poem is a prayer,
a down payment on faith.

If there were no Fifth Floor,
where would the children be?
Where else could I learn
about *holding on*—

and *letting go*—
but on the Fifth Floor,
at the center
of the universe.

THE GOD OF BROKEN THINGS
after Yusef Komunyakaa

This ancient god reincarnates
dearly departed toys and treasures,
the movement of his wrinkled hands
angel-wing smooth
as he saves the unsalvageable,

gluing, rasping, repairing in his basement kingdom
of twisted twine, bent brass, knickknacks, bric-a-bracs,
awash in the acrid incense
of smoldering solder, serenaded by
a heavenly choir of children laughing.

The masked minor god, gowned in sky-blue
surgical scrubs, tinkers with
broken bodies, repairing the ravages
of delinquent diets, splintered genes, sins
of omission and commission.

He conjures up his usual lesser-miracle,
one he can do in his sleep, or with no sleep,
guiding the tube through the maze of arteries,
simple as piloting the Sun's chariot
from dawn to dusk.

Maybe it's karma, kismet,
fate, fatigue, or faulty stopcock
that allows the freckle-sized bubble of air
to slip from the tip of the catheter,
and in the cathedral quiet of the surgical suite

he gasps, reaches a gloved hand to the image
on the TV screen, watches the ascension
to the brain,
surprise in the old man's eyes
at the dawning of the stroke.

Now unmasked, the minor god
watches bubbles drift up the neck
of his beer bottle, awaits amnesia,
anesthesia, the cries of children
effervescing from the surface

of his psyche, barely obscured
by the blare of the jukebox.

Good Friday at the Art Museum

Caught in the eye of the brush,
Mary sits at his limp right hand,
cradles his head,
the burial shroud at her feet.

Torchlight flickers placenta-red
off eyes rolled toward
the bruised-plum heavens,
an indifferent Ohio sky.

This isn't Michelangelo's Pietà
hung in the town of Oberlin,
but one by a nameless
eighteenth century Italian.

Stains on her cloak suggest
the paint has been retouched,
or are those teardrops?
If you stand just right, you glimpse

a hint of her halo, though
she doesn't look blessed
as she plucks thorns from his scalp,
washes dried blood from wounds

she could not prevent,
wounds more painful than childbirth,
her last embrace held for the same eternity
it took your blue shirt

to convert to a deep wine,
bathed in your blood, as I held you,
waiting for you to move,
to say *Mother*.

LIFE

What a strange machine man is! You fill him with bread, wine, fish, and radishes, and out comes sighs, laughter, and dreams.
—Nikos Kazantzakis

Living Color

I walked out on childhood
in tennis shoes, which like TVs,
came solely in black and white.
Kids wore *Keds*
only for sports and only on courts—
before *Nike* shuffled sneakers
into nursing homes, flubbered them
into high-rise offices.
I spray painted mine
screaming Day-Glo red and green,
then boogaloo'd through a monochrome world
about to be tie-dyed.

Now, uniformed in business drab,
pinstriped seasons swirl me
to meetings and deadlines
on thin-soled wingtips
which no longer catch the breeze.
How curious to find a life
lost in this dusty shoebox,
dormant until now—
as if called by need.

Sea Shell

Your brine-hardened back
is arched against a ruthless world,
yet firelight seeps through scars,
gouges chiseled on careless days.

I recognize our brotherhood—
marooned vagabonds
who both prefer liberty
to the shelter of the coral reef.

Your black etched grooves
show scrimshaw character,
like dirty fingernails or the wrinkles
at the corners of my eyes.

Ivory ridges stand in relief,
square as teeth
smiling along your edge,
a seafarer's shore-leave grin.

My fingernails strum
while you return
a syncopated,
washboard rhythm.

Surging wave riffs and seabird laments
join our makeshift reggae band,
as I wail the blues rock steady,
sipping moonlight and rum.

Brown Anole

From the shade of yaupon shrubs
and sable palms, a brown anole
joins me in the Florida sun, both of us
solar-powered, recharging.

The lizard's not interested until
I turn a page in my book.
He cocks his head, fixes me
with a cold, dark eye—

for movement means a meal, life.
He lassos a passing ant with his tongue,
licks his lips, stares at the sun, then at me,
waits for global warming,

for climate change, like the last time
when cousin T-Rex relinquished the kingdom.
With brainstem bravado, he balloons his neck,
pistons up and down

doing pushups with toothpick arms,
pumping up for the day
the earth's axis shifts
again.

Between
a tanka

Silver fish frozen
in blue ice, midway between
lake and sky, between
yesterday and tomorrow,
between harsh winter and spring.

Rice Paper Seasons
haiku series

Spring:
Sparrows erratic
shadows mirror through water
the movement of fish,

as rice paper wings
carry them far from our own
linear world.

Summer:
My hammock, roofed by
leaves and bird song, along side
a spider's hammock,

the lake in silken
gown dancing with pinstriped birch
'neath a lantern moon.

Autumn:
Crows high on corn mash
play follow-the-leader like
roller coaster cars,

then hide-n-seek with
field mice scampering through
dry cornstalk stubble.

Winter:
Black birds on white snow
call to their city cousins -
white birds on black snow,

while I, in my loft,
write life snippets, as ravens
tap at my window.

BLACKBIRD

Raindrops plump as seedless grapes
spatter the pavement, batter the roof, as I
enter the haven of *The Leeward Lounge*.
Egan squats on his usual stool, drops a depth-charge
of his friend, *Jim Beam*, into his beer,
caresses his *Marlboro*, stares at the deaf-mute
TV, talks politics, dirty tricks.

Outside the alley window, backlit by a streetlamp,
a dark figure flips a coin,
sets it on the sill,
cocks his head, looks straight at me
like some street punk—then taps the pane,
bobs his head, picks up the coin
in his beak, flips it again.

A door slams; I await the arrival
of the late, great Mr. Poe,
but it's Egan, not Edgar,
back from the john.
He glances at the window, says
*In the old country, a bird at the window
means death*, then segues to lawn care.

The other stool-toppers look, but do not see.
As the jukebox flat-lines, the bird
taps out an urgent rhythm.
I half-expect him to spit in the street, light a stogie,
sell me tout sheets or tiny Rolex knockoffs
hidden under feathers, but he
just keeps flipping: heads, tails, heads.

What does he want? I wonder
if he's warning or threatening,
but like Egan's chatter, there is no end.
Maybe he's laying odds on my demise:
if it's tails, will my neon-red life
drain from my veins, mix with spilled beer
on the peanut-shelled floor until

I fade into the night, as black as he.
Mayhem taps again on the window.
A cackle erupts, yet he's not smiling.
A drop, too dark for rain,
trickles down the pane.
As Egan rambles on about dental care
through yellowed teeth, I pocket

happy-hour nuts, pay the barkeep.
Outside, I raise my collar,
enter the alley, but he's gone.
I stare at blood on the window,
the tail-side of a penny on the sill,
trade peanuts for the coin, payment
for advice given, time spent.

Today in church, I long
to fly home, long for *Jim Beam*
to ease the scratch
of gravel in my throat, yet
tuck the penny under the coffin pillow,
plod the stairs to the podium,
croon my short elegy for Egan, my heart

fluttering
like the beating
of black wings.

In Another Time

we'd sit by the fire, your hair
cascading to your hips,
the baby at your breast,
both of you wrapped in coats
of beasts I killed with sharp stones

a million sunsets ago,
shrieks of survival slicing night air
black as the cave—
the gash on my thigh
oozing thick yellow-green.

Or I'd be sprawled on the settee, the memory
of smoked ham and cornbread in the air,
the last log sizzling in the stove by the crib,
ribbons painting my uniform with rainbows
of glory won in some skirmish for Napoleon,

Lincoln, or Lee—a musket ball
lodged in my side—as you
fetch blankets, hot tea laced
with honeyed whiskey, your lips
miming every prayer you know.

Instead, I lie in a gown of white
on a bed of white, you slumped in a chair,
humming a lullaby for baby and me
to the metronome beat
of dripping saline, the EKG

ticking like our grandfather clock
when it needs winding.
No furs. No flags.
No meat. No medals.
Just the ticking, the dripping,

the taste of poisons, unanswered questions.
Just this army of angry cells
torching the countryside,
breaching the barricades, the ending
always the same.

Positive

        Nothing in his closet.
Like two peas in a perverted pod—
him and his heathen friend!
        She disembowels his backpack,
        palpates the extruded contents.
Hang with white trash fags with AIDS
and you get no privacy, boy!
        Her searchlight scatters
        dust bunnies under the bed.
Damn apple didn't fall far
from his Daddy's kinky tree!
        She hunkers down
        with the laundry basket,
        launches a rainbow
        of dirty clothes
        like a roman candle.
I better not find
pictures of boys!
        The dresser drawer rains down
        on the swell of teen treasures
        that overflows his bed,
        as sunlight reflects golden
        off a condom wrapper.
Damn!
I knew it!
        She mine sweeps the sock drawer,
        brings up loose change and Lifesavers.
I give him life—
what's he give me?
        She gropes through tattered t-shirts
        and dingy shorts until
        fire ignites in her palm,
        the syringe clinging
        to her retreating hand
        like a viper
        with a barbed metal fang—
        as blood brooks flow
        through fields of flesh
        and the warm dawn
        awakens death threads of DNA, destined
        to breed the answer
        to her question.

The Tough Trek Home

From my dark basement corner, I half-expect
Dante to descend the stairs
as I read the braille
of battered lives.
Brutish truth shuffles by in scuffed shoes.

Folding chairs and folded lives,
cold and hard, creak
as they start to unfold again,
heads bowed in prayer, resignation
or acceptance.

Fred combs yellowed fingers
through remembered hair,
his belly the size
of the kegs of beer
he's chugged for years.

Dan is drunk again on frosted jiggers
of self-pity.
Rose, our resident arsonist,
lights bonfires
of cigarettes and prayer candles.

I do the twelve step shuffle
through the fluorescent flicker
and hum of discontent,
tap the microphone, say
Hi, my name is Nora…

while outside the window,
feral need howls like coyotes
calling my name, reminding me
it's a short stroll from Eden to Babylon,
but a tough trek home.

Hindsight

My ancient Harley shudders
over potholes and concrete clefts,
but that's not why my hands shake.
      Death smiles toothless
        in my rearview mirror, smokes
          a stogie, eyes me like a bird of prey.
His bulldog hood-ornament nips at my
jet-streamed hair, snarls at the peace symbol
on my jacket, growls a foot from my fender.

He shoves me toward the bumper sticker
of the truck ahead that reads *Love America
or Leave It*—maybe in a body bag.
      The tattooed nude on his arm CBs
      the third truck blocking the passing lane, says
      We got us a funeral convoy.
Escape and the rough road to hell
are both paved with gravel
in an unsoft shoulder.

Sunlight sparkles on my balding front tire
and I hear Jim Morrison sing
This Is The End.
      The trucks spit stones. I smell tar,
      taste blood as red
      lights flash, hear the wail
drop an octave as an ambulance
sweeps the truck from the high-speed lane,
and the waters part.

I lean hard into the curve,
    nearly fuse with my shadow,
        hear my beast howl as I twist
           the throttle, the wind
              like a fist in my face.
                I wedge behind the siren,
                    shout over my shoulder, the words
                    and spittle stretching thin—
                      then goose the engine and go,

                            one eye forever
                            on the rearview.

SILENCE

Silence is reticent, reflective,
reserves judgment,
holds its tongue.

It's the unspoken anger of a wife,
the frown of her husband, their child
listening from the top of the stairs.

Only monks, martyrs, poets,
and those whose needs are small
willingly pay its price.

Yet, meditation is not solitude
but a gathering with God, a silent
celebration of birth, life, death.

Silence can also sprout in the cracks
between piano keys, flourish amid notes,
bloom in the rhythm

of the poet's pen, each thought
alive in the white space
between lines and stanzas

where everything
is said
without words.

Matthew 5:49 (The B- Attitudes)
"I will accept no bull from your house" (Psalms 50:9)

>Blessed are the quick
>to dawdle and dream,
>those who listen to the sound
>of their thoughts,
>>for they shall linger over lattes
>>and be called *Poets.*
>
>Blessed are the piece-makers
>with deadlines,
>writers who toil against time,
>>for they shall be called the children
>>of desperation.
>
>Blessed are the blank
>of mind and page,
>>for theirs is the kingdom
>>of possibility.
>
>Blessed are they who suffer persecution
>for publication sake,
>>for they shall find comfort
>>in Prozac.
>
>Blessed are those with prodigal
>fingers wandering the keyboard desert,
>>for He[1] shall provide
>>spell-checker.
>
>Blessed are the poor of shekels,
>whose ledgers fill with red ink,
>content with a tome in one hand,
>cheap wine in the other,
>>for they shall render
>>stones unto the tax collector.
>
>And blessed are the meek
>lovers who intone
>with minimal scorn:
>*Silence, the poet works!*
>>for they shall inherit
>>the housework.

[1] Bill Gates

Finding the Words

Hop on the highway to exit 8,
turn right on the third dirt road
until the brook's bright babble becomes
a waterfall's roar at the beaver dam.

There you'll find the wild words,
feral critters with teeth and claws to slash
the humdrum from your first draft,
startle your readers, and even yourself.

Or head downtown to the beat
of horns and traffic, past ripe dumpsters,
to back alleys and pool halls
where street words hang out.

Jaw with the folks, score some
vintage doo-wop, or pocket a baggie
of the latest urban hip
to spice up your poetry stew.

There's a place in the foothills
where lyrical words roam free as mustangs,
so lively and lithe they're tough to corral,
though with practice you'll rope a few.

Can't help you with the three-piece formal verse
because I gave up suits and ties, though I suspect
you still can kidnap a couple stanzas
from Ivy League class reunions and trendy cigar bars.

Or just do what I do—drink wine with the Muse,
pretend to write while swaying in sunset currents,
then wade hip-deep into rivers of stars
and pan your dreams for glittering nuggets.

Essence

To sculpt marble metaphors
    That weather time—

To dance without music
    Yet twirl to new rhythms—

To whittle away remnants
    Revealing the image within—

To paint without pigment
    Yet gild the landscape—

To weave warmth without a loom
    Inching line by thread—

To bring life to a boil
    Distilling its essential oils—

To spin gossamer webs
    Alive with stinging spiders—

To strike pen upon paper
    Then weld with the flame—

To create whirlwinds
    With the final draft—

To sing thoughts a cappella
    While a stranger begins

To hum the harmony
    Of poetry's timeless duet.

Generic Novel

My soon-to-be bestselling novel,
which I've not yet begun, should open
with mist veiling an island, because clues
always wash onshore from your left
as you circle the beach clockwise
pondering enigmas.

Our hero, let's call him Lance or Buck, will be
like me, but with less gray hair and no need for pants
with Magic-Stretch waistbands.
He'll be powerful as his Lear Jet,
flashy as his Lamborghini, captivating
the female demographic.
Of course, I'll delete any mention
of wrinkles, bifocals, or hemorrhoids.

He'll need a love interest, a challenging woman,
every bit his match, yet a little lusty and lost.
Let's make her two decades younger, though—
Trust me on this! I'm a professional!—
the reader will never notice, because our hero
will be a geezer-jock, surfing big breakers,
dunking balls through hoops.

Their dialog will be a web of snappy repartee,
except for the scene in a sidewalk café
when Buck professes his love, while she
silently sips her decaf latte, unable to meet his gaze—
which should be easy for me to write.

Our villain must be more devious
than IRS agents, more diabolical
than even a mother-in-law.
I'll pepper the narrative with gunfire,
car chases, betrayal, the usual mayhem, until
our heroes prevail, and Buck hoists his love
into the dry-dock of his arms,
carries her to their hut on the beach,
where they'll live happily ever after
awaiting my next unwritten novel—while I
sip wine, nibble cheese at writers' workshops,
pontificating about *process* and *craft*.

My Muse

Come hither ye atheists, Christians, and Jews
and gather ye writers from whom the words ooze.
Come brethren who freely a lifetime pay dues,
for whom "mental block" is yesterday's news.
Those o'er the abyss, who oft sing the blues,
who frequent the depths with nothing to lose,
assemble your courage and summon your muse.

(insert whistle here, as if hailing a cab)

Then from ether spring images,
some singular or in twos,
bright multicolored visions
in unique shapes and hues,
clear eloquent thoughts,
vivid ideas to use,
until from your soul
great literature spews.

But now in reflection this poem I peruse,
my valiant attempt is naught but a ruse.
The muse on *my* shoulder must be hittin' the booze!

Ode to Glory

Don't pity my peculiar limp,
sliding every fourth step.
Injuries are the price of glory.

This trophy case once proclaimed
we were the best in Cleveland,
all-American boys in an all-American sport.

We played without helmets or pads,
with a ball too heavy to throw,
too dangerous to catch.

Grim-faced gladiators in powder-blue uniforms,
we marched in shoes of many colors
through a haze of Old Spice and Lucky Strikes

past the Dirty Harry pinball machine
to the strains of "Leader of the Pack"
and applause from the folks at the bar.

I hung tough as scarlet oozed from my lip
and a trickle of ketchup
stained the name on my shirt pocket.

We brought home the gold-
painted statue on the plastic stand, confirming
we were the best damn team

no one ever heard of.
The guys who always
never got the girls.

So, after I'm gone, in my memory
lay a six-pack and a carton of smokes
at the tomb of this unknown bowler.

RESERVATIONS
penned on a greasy napkin

On the south shore of Sandusky Bay, perch
school-up at the corner of Main and Market
on the walls of the Lake Erie Diner.

The room fills with secondhand smoke,
grease-spatter, and a medley
of fishermen, Village People,

and Jimmy Buffett wannabes,
whose backsides overflow
the memory dents

molded in the naugahyde seats
by smaller generations.
In a photo on the wall,

someone's grandfather
kisses a catfish.
Christmas lights blink in the window

and a stuffed Easter Bunny's button
says *Welcome Spring*, though
it's July and ninety degrees in here.

Our waitress, a charm school
dropout, wipes our table with a gym sock,
sweats out our orders like confessions—

then belts them like Janis Joplin
to the backbeat of wire brushes
on the grill and silverware cymbals.

The harried cook, singing backup
in an accent I can't quite place,
stands below a *Kwitcherbelliakin* sign.

Yet my belly doesn't ache
until he bare-hands my Zeus burger,
coughs on my side of cabbage, and I recall

this joint is only one block from the Eternal Light
Funeral Home, specializing in *pre-planned services*—
and I wonder if I should have planned ahead.

The World's Sexiest Man

Attracted by a feeding frenzy of females
at the grocery store magazine rack, I find
TV Guide featuring full-color photos
of *The World's Sexiest Men*—yet strangely,
my picture is not among them.

The man on the cover hasn't shaved in days,
may not have bathed, wears a rumpled coat
of dead animal skin over a black PETA t-shirt,
his boxer's nose angled beneath ice-blue eyes
that could freeze warts.

Clearly, this man is a handywoman's dream,
a few minor projects from perfection. The caption reads:
Great body. Damn fine hair. And a brain surgeon!
on TV—though I suspect his stringless guitar
is a metaphor for his soul.

But he's finished second to a shirtless guy, chest gilded
by golden curls, who's apparently affixed to the page
by a large piercing through his navel. I'm sure he speaks
European suave in an FM bass so deep
it would rattle Grandma's dentures,

and if you brought him home to meet Mom,
you can bet he'd hit on her.
Somehow, he manages to swagger
as he slouches, legs spread, wearing torn blue jeans,
a smirk that says: *No boxers. No briefs.*

Back home, I share the joke with my lover, yet
there is no laughter as she thumbs the photos,
concentrates as if reading Chekhov.
Then, without looking up, she says: *Honey,
you should shower and shave,*

as she heads for our bedroom—
and suddenly I feel like
The World's Sexiest Man.

Marilyn, What Is It Like

to walk into a party
all skin and sin and grins,
eyelids at half-mast, red tongue
bisecting white teeth, and watch
a room full of mouths
open but empty of sound;

to have the power to say *no*—knowing,
like a magician, you could always pull a *yes*
from your fashionable, wide-brim hat,
easy as flipping a light switch
with a hot-pink, polished pinky,
turning lovers from *off* to *on*;

to make it day or night
for someone else
because you decide to sleep,
sleep around, not sleep at all;
to spin in powerful circles
with Jack, Joe, Marlon,

a glass of Dom Pérignon,
pot, or pills always a whim away,
free to do anything, nothing, the world
your oyster, caviar, Lafite Rothschild;
to know the laws of physics,
economics, society, gravity

don't apply to you, that you
are only ruled by the laws
of heavenly bodies,
soaring among the stars
'til life becomes so blasé
you just stop flapping your wings.

Jesus Left Me Today

He walked out of my life, said
there was no saving me
from me, that I could go to hell
if I wanted, because eternity
was too damn short and he
wouldn't dangle from my cross.

He told me he was tired of feeling invisible,
of bringing home the daily bread
without so much as a *howdy-do,*
said it was time to get out
of the wheel barrel and push, to find
my way in this world and the next.

When he cleaned out his closet,
the fridge, my last carton of Kools,
I said, *Hey lamb, don't leave.*
He said if I wanted to see him, I could
put down my Hostess Twinkies,
turn off Jerry Springer, and go to his place.

Said he was getting off the bus,
gum on the seats, windows stuck shut,
everyone looking one direction,
riding in circles for forever, then
he grabbed a bottle of Manischewitz,
a good book, flipped on his shades,

and walked out the door,
hitching a ride toward Bethlehem, PA
until he was in the wind.

Snapshots at a Wedding

Spent rain ponds   on a rented limo.

    She checks her watch, a ticking
    time bomb between age spots.
    Wife or Life? she wonders.

Potted palms   shade them like umbrellas.

    His face is frosted glass, so pale
    the girls in his dreams
    can't see him.

The bride and groom smile   atop the cake,

    behind them, winding rivers
    of soot and ash, memories
    of incinerated dreams.

Charcoal birds   checkmark a pastel sun.

    They stand at the zero,
    where numbers and lives
    either surge or shrivel.

White roses   wilt on a weathered trellis.

    They exchange rings
    but not glances, wrap their arms
    like ropes around their brokenness.

Waves weep upon sand,   then disappear.

Seasoned Citizens:
Thirteen Ways of Looking at Gray Birds
with apologies to Wallace Stevens and to blackbirds

I
Among the snowy graves
of four dead husbands, the widow
vows to marry again and complete
her six-pack plot.

II
I am of three colors:
canary-yellow shirt, lime-green pants,
matching white belt and shoes.

III
Her wrinkled hands whirl in the autumn winds.
Her husband enjoys the pantomime
of quiet time together,
his hearing aid turned off.

IV
Though a man and his Cadillac are one,
at fifteen miles per hour, no deer need fear.
Yet a man, his Cadillac, and a three-legged squirrel
are also one.

V
I do not know which to prefer:
endless sexual innuendo or Viagra,
with Biff and Buffy blissfully boffing
between pinochle and shuffle board.

VI
Images fill the tinted windshield: a Lilliputian
perched on a phone book, blue hair
peeking over the wheel, the pedals
barely within reach.

VII
Oh old men of Sun City,
players of eight-track tapes,
why, in your Golden Years, do you imagine
young, golden chicks?
Do you not see that you are
the few surviving roosters
among a multitude of hens?

VIII
I know the noble penny
and the lucid, inescapable rhythms
of compound interest; but I also know
my children share my fascination
with my savings account.

IX
When the tires finally come to rest
on the sidewalk, the hem of her dress
still flapping outside the driver's door,
this marks the end of many circles
around the parking lot.

X
At the sight of the elderly couple
stopped at a green light
long enough to read *War and Peace*,
even the heavily-sedated
would cry out sharply.

XI
He once road showroom-bright over Connecticut,
but after replacement of valves
and hips, he takes solace in his grill
of original teeth,
and though no longer in running condition,
he still walks well.

XII
The old man is moving forward.
His turn signal blinks *left*
until the bulb burns out.

XIII
There is no rush in *rush hour*
when you live in another time zone,
another dimension where it's today
all day long,
and early bird dinner starts at four,
bedtime at dusk.

Worship

When the world is asleep
or at Sunday service,
she steps off the mountain
looking for God and He

embraces her
in thermal eddies,
lifts her like a mirage
above arroyos, cacti and sage.

Having found the purple apparel
and floppy red hat of old age wanting,
she chooses a pink helmet and prone position
in hang gliding, as in life.

She sings His glory
with every updraft,
hovers where each moment
is Judgment Day,

ascends into tickless time
where the only sound is wind
blowing life into her lungs,
exhales her refrain:

*Thy will be done on earth
as it is this high above*—then,
touches down, roof-racks her glider, begins
the slow migration to early-bird dinner,

leaving the heavens
and the bunny hills
to the church-blessed
and Sunday hangovers.

Ageless

God, she loves the feel
of fine leather on soft skin,
the sinuous whip
of wind, the bore and stroke,
the throaty purr as she
wraps her legs around

her Softail Fat Boy.
Together, they are
two-tone, pink on ebony,
hot as dual exhausts,
driven by the throb
of Twin Cam 88s.

The smile she gives the boys
in the Ford pickup says
*My silver hair has seen
more than you can dream,*
as she milks the throttle, leaves them
back home where they belong.

Wrapped in a consensual breeze,
she watches her odometer ratchet up,
peers in the teardrop rearview
remembering past rides, knowing
the road ends around some bend.
But she's a street poet, so she

listens to the rhythm
of tires on concrete,
weaves through line breaks
on the road and in her mind,
her saddlebags filled
with yesterdays,

with room for tomorrow—then
she gooses her Hog, thinks:
Now that's poetry!

Softail Fat Boy motorcycles are the exclusive trademark of the Harley-Davidson Motor Co.
Ford is the exclusive trademark of The Ford Motor Company.
Hogs just are.

Feeling Invisible
a middle-age limerick

There once was a confident older gent
who figured his youth was inherent.
But young girls passed him by
without blinking an eye
'til he realized he was transparent!

Hangin' with Grandma

There, in a tree, my grandma is hangin'…
strung up like a bad B western.
No tunnel of light,
no choir of angels.

Kickin' and twitchin'
and utterin' a string
of discouraging words
that would make a sailor blush

pink as her jumpsuit,
she waits for the cavalry
in the chase car
under an orange nylon sky.

A renewable source of chutzpah
happy to still be hangin' around,
she unhitches her harness,
drops like Newton's apple

jackboots to the ground
from a cottonwood nearly her age,
hoping an elderly body in motion
will stay in motion.

Last year, divin' oceans. Today, divin' skies.
Next birthday, who knows?
Rock climbin' or rugby?—*anything*
but the rockin' chair.

Downhill

It's a jailbreak of sorts,
from the assisted living center
to the airport.

She laughs when the metal-detector
rats out her hip-prosthesis
and hip-flask of bourbon,

smiles when they search her shoes,
says her only explosives
are in her colon.

No time for tans, she
slips a Hawaiian shirt
over sports bra and bike pants,

flips down her state-cop shades,
and leaps from plane
to taxi, arriving at the summit

as wine-colored first light
pours down the goblet
of Haleakala Crater.

A Polynesian sun god
answers her prayer;
bronze hands raise her

onto a bike, her cane
deadwood on the ground.
With zinc oxide, he

whites out her nose, paper-tapes
GRANDMA on her helmet, says
Follow me.

Amid stillness and moonbows,
ten fledgling riders
swoop down miles of switchbacks

toward the sea
like pelicans in a row.
Silver hair streaming, she rides gravity

into cloud-tops,
lingers there
tasting heaven

'til their helmets pour out
like multicolored rain
down the mountain.

She coasts her borrowed youth
to sand's edge, where
this small dormant volcano,

at the base of the largest, erupts
in giggles, accepts a Lohelani flower
and hug from the sun god, then

whispers what she always whispers
to any god who will listen:
Mahalo.

---

* *Mahalo* is the Hawaiian word for "Thank you."

Sepia World

Wrapped in a patchwork quilt
of yesterdays, she flips through her youth,
reviews her life in slow-motion,
frame by frame, each sepia photo
a butterfly memory pinned to the page.

She visits her family. Papa
in his suit and suspenders, back stiff
as the chair he sits on, restless hands
holding each other in his lap, his face
grim because the world was.
Ma, round and doughy, stands behind him,
a steady hand on his shoulder, eyes fixed
somewhere in Europe, motionless
as dead family.

In another, fresh flowers planted
in hand painted vases surround
an early edition of herself, gift-wrapped
in a crinoline skirt and hair ribbon bows.
She smiles, cradles her baby brother,
dressed in his christening gown, not knowing
his photo will soon be followed
by his prayer card.

Then one of the old neighborhood, porches lined
with extra chairs reserved for neighbors
with the same accent, friends
emerging like new world weeds
through concrete cracks.
And in the corner store, eggs
float in vats of pickle juice, and flies
single-file through screen holes, lining up
on strips of sticky paper
hung from the ceiling.

In one with a tattered edge torn away
like a corner of Nebraska,
she sits on the sofa at sixteen, her knees
two sentries guarding frilled bloomers—
and even today, she can still smell
the blue-black smoke of the coal furnace, see
paper boats racing down Woodland Boulevard
in rainwater rivers, feel the warmth of summer nights
lit by lightening bugs in Mason jars, taste the dandelion wine
lips of pimple-faced boys kissed under oil-lit streetlamps.

She closes her sepia world, returns the album
to the wicker trunk with black metal hinges,
A. Petera, Cleveland O.
painted in bright green on its top—
a name changed to *Peters*
by some nameless clerk at Ellis Island
when it wouldn't dance
with his Yankee tongue; an address
meant for a lifetime.

OBERLIN
after Carl Sandburg

    Bigotry Butcher for the World,
    Book and Music Maker, Stacker of Corn,
    Builder of Invisible Railroads and Precious Cargo Handler;
    Scrappy, wiry, peacemaker,
    Town of Big Conscience:

They tell me you are hayseed and I believe them, for I
    have seen your farmers' markets,
    your dollar movie shows.

And they tell me you are quick to anger and I answer: Yes, it is true,
    I have seen the other cheek turn
    red with rage at the sight of injustice.

And they tell me you are not rich and my reply is: Wealth has colors
    other than gold and green.

And having answered so, I turn once more to those who
    sneer at this, my town, and give them back the sneer
    and say to them:

Come and show me another town where train tracks pierce the earth
    from history, tyranny, bondage, the whip, emerging
    like a drowning man, sucking in all the freedom he can hold.

Come and show me another town built on the rich soil
    of righteousness, where Century homes have secret rooms
    connected to underground tunnels and liberty.

Come and show me another town that escorted women
    and men of all colors from cornfields and kitchens
    to classrooms and corporations.

Come and show me another town where the intersection
    of Main Street and College really is, where music and ideas
    float on the breeze from open windows.

Flinging viscous curses amid the toil of piling truth on right,
    here is a sinewy scarred grappler, wrestling
    with issues, unbowed before big soft cities;

Fierce when faced with a bloodhound's fangs, cunning
     as a slave pitted against the wilderness,

          Town-gowned,
          Contemplating,
          Communicating,
          Composing,
          Creating, breaking, remaking,

Under torch smoke of the Oberlin-Wellington Rescue,
     white teeth laughing through blood-crusted lips,
Under the terrible burden of destiny laughing
     as a wise man laughs,
Laughing even as a fighter laughs who fears
     neither fist nor foe,
Bragging and laughing that under his ribs,
     beats the pulse of the people,

          Laughing!

Laughing the stormy, wiry, scrappy laughter of a Peacemaker,
     unafraid of the fray, bare-chested, sweating, proud to be

          Bigotry Butcher, Book and Music Maker,
          Stacker of Corn, Builder of Invisible Railroads
          and Precious Cargo Handler to the Nation.

GEORGIA O'KEEFFE—A FOUND POEM

*It is what I have done with where I have been
that should be of interest.*
—Georgia O'Keeffe

Budding like a *Pink Sweet Pea*
in a pasture of wine-stained prairie grass,
a farmer's seedling, first cousin
of the soil, your fate was sealed.

Dressed in *Black Iris* clothing,
wide-eyed as *Belladonna*, you sprouted notions
crazy as *Jimson Weed*, became bilingual
in color and texture, painted poems
of things unnoticed.

With no Monet, the world
disinherited the meek
flowers, until you
grew them wall-sized, zoomed in so we
could caress their sensual soft parts,
hung like Art Deco lamps,
addicting as *Nicotina*.

For a time, you dabbled in the colors
of sin, a *Spotted Lily*,
letting the camera paint you
wearing only a derby and a grin,
as natural as a *Red Poppy*,
while you reveled in life
close to the eye:
dewdrops on petals,
the occasional insect,
blemish, body hair.

Then you fled the lens, drawn like a lover
to the fickle palette of southwestern sky, embraced
the wonderful emptiness,
rooted deep in the desert,
tasted the sweet pain
as the Palo Duro Canyon
slashed the plains, felt the heat
of underground springs,
not unlike your own.

You polished your grandmother's
pioneer spirit, pumped water,
learned to ride, to shoot,
shoveled rattlers from your old adobe,
not far from the atomic womb
of Los Alamos, where you painted
the *Black Cross* on a crimson horizon,
White Calico Flowers awaiting graves.

You lived in a world of charcoal and oils,
of moist life and dry death, discovered
the *Cup of Silver* the conquistadors sought,
unearthed the American spirit
where the spirits of Native Americans roam.
And when the *Calico Roses* blossomed
in the steer's skull,
the *White Trumpet Flower* played
a national anthem so distinctive
it needed no lyrics.

Although you wished upon canvas
all things loved,
buttes, rivers, barns,
even a *New York Night*,
now that your bones
bleach in the desert heat,
it is your flowers,
scattered like children
you never had,
that carry on your family name—
a lineage of
Miracle Flowers
in perennial bloom.

---

* The titles of fourteen O'Keeffe paintings are highlighted in italics.

When I Dreamt of Daughters

I expected honey and spice,
    pirouettes and puppies,
    stuffed bunnies and bears, not
    boogers and pet mice.

I envisioned tiny violins, but never
    a trombone, taller and more brassy
    even than you—then thanked God
    when you settled on piano.

I told bedtime stories,
    you told fairytales
    about your brother
    shoving you down the stairs.

I anticipated stylish salons and silk gowns,
    not jumbo pink eyeglasses,
    or mushroom clouds
    of Orphan Annie curls.

I foresaw skinned knees, understood that some
    reassembly might be required,
    but never anticipated
    appendicitis at age eight.

I relished your giggles and grins,
    shining through untamed teeth
    corraled by braces—
    worth every penny when you smile.

I bought dollhouses and jump ropes
    that collected dust, while you
    went downhill skiing
    and climbed rock walls.

I awaited questions, got opinions—
    watched your resolve
    blossom into three point shots,
    four point grades.

I perused finger paintings and crayon doodles
    long before I understood beauty—yet,
    as you stand at the altar, I'm certain
    Michelangelo would weep.

So, dear daughter, walk boldly
    into the dawn of this new love
    you've searched for
    all your life,

and begin your future together,
    once and forever,
    as two reflections
    in the same silvered mirror.

Grail

Heft it. Feel its weight.
Swirl the nectar, release the bouquet
of charred oak, hints of coffee, cloves.
It is time.
Take your first sip
from the Holy Grail.
I pass it on to you, my child.

It is your birthright, blessing, burden—
not because you're the most holy, it's just
that you're descended from servants
who cleared tables
a hundred generations ago,
born to a family of vintners, stewards
of more than wine.

You might expect a glow, an aura,
a rim of rubies, the shimmer
of sapphires,
a cipher of ancient symbols
that answers all questions—
but it's just
a humble metal cup.

Yet even chardonnay, aged for an instant
in this vessel, transforms
to the garnet hue of a deep bruise,
the flavor complex, layered
with ample almond, earth, plum,
the subtle teeth of tannins
nibbling the tongue like a lover,

the fruit, acid and sugars as balanced
as a life well lived, the body
weighing on the palate like velvet,
the finish everlasting, lingering
like a sustained symphonic chord.
Let your mouth become a chalice,
each sip a kind of faith

that the sun is our communion wafer, the moon
a host of reflected love, the glow within you
divine revelation.
For in this goblet, wine is not a beverage
but the grape gone heavenly,
released from bondage, as we all shall be
released from *our* skin.

Remember, this cup was full
long before the Bible,
before the thought
of rain on a grape seed.
It was crafted to fit the hand,
to serve.
Savor, my child.

Taste.
Share.
May its very existence
remove the nails
from your daily cross
as it has from mine
for a lifetime.

ACKNOWLEDGMENTS CONTINUED:

The Penwood Review: "Monsters and Ghosts"
Tattoo Highway: "A Miss America Pageant Finalist" (originally titled "Beached")
The LLI Review: "Bordeaux Simple" and "The Tough Trek Home"
Soundings Review: "Mr. Fix-It"
Slant: "Mood Music"
The Fourth River: "Constant"
Natural Bridge: "Another Found Poem" and "Chains"
Common Threads: "September Bloom," "Shrapnel" (originally titled "Sunday Morning, Nine AM"), and "Positive"
The Litchfield Review: "Portable Memories"
This Hard Wind: "Rocks"
Words of Comfort, Words of Courage (Australia): "Manhattan Streets"
The Vincent Brothers Review: "Glass of Absinthe" and "Extra Innings"
Sandhill Review: "Twenty-One Gun Tanka"
The Kerf: "Bedside"
Journal of the American Medical Association: 2002, 288:1562, ©2002, American Medical Association. All Rights reserved: "The Unbearable Weight of Ashes"
Pebble Lake Review: "Sea Shell"
Ellipsis: "Brown Anole"
Tanka Splendor 2003: "Between" (originally titled "Silver Fish")
First Person Pleural: "Matthew 5:49"
HA! Magazine: "My Muse"
Bowling Digest: "Ode to Glory"
Clare: "Worship"
Biker Ally—The Motorcycle Magazine Geared For Women: "Ageless"
Encore 2004—Prize Poems of the National Federation of State Poetry Societies: "Hangin' with Grandma"
Tar Wolf Review—A Journal of Poetry and Art: "Georgia O'Keeffe—A Found Poem"

POEM AWARDS
"The People's Republic" was inducted in 2002 into the permanent collection of the George Bush Presidential Library, and reprinted in *Red, White and Blues: Poets on the Promise of America* by the University of Iowa Press.
"Appetites" was awarded 1st Prize in Poetry by *Ascent Aspirations Magazine* (Canada).
"Black and White Photograph" was awarded 1st Place in the New Words 2008 Poetry Competition (The Akron Art Museum).

"Permanent Record," "Worship," and "Waltzing with Roethke" were awarded 1st Place in the 14th Annual Lorain County Community College Literary Festival.

"A Miss America Pageant Finalist" was awarded Best Poem in the A Picture Worth 500 Words Contest (Creative Writing Program of California State University, Hayward).

"Positive" was awarded 1st Place in the 2002 TOCOPA Poetry Contest (sponsored by the Tiffin Area Chapter of the Ohio Poetry Association).

"Sea Shell" was awarded 1st Place in the 2nd Annual Rising Sun Poetry Competition (*Rising Sun Magazine*).

"September Bloom" was awarded 1st Place in the 2002 Summer Solstice Contest (The Ohio Poetry Association).

"Shrapnel" (originally titled "Sunday Morning, Nine AM") was awarded 1st Place in the 2002 Vernal Equinox Contest (The Ohio Poetry Association).

About The Author

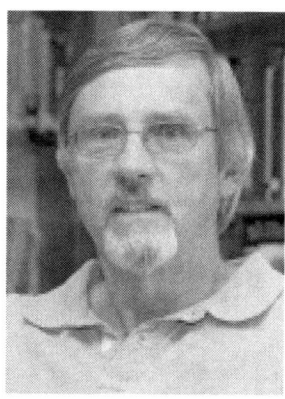

John (Jack) Vanek was born and raised in the Cleveland, Ohio area. He received his bachelor's degree from Case Western Reserve University, where his passion for creative writing took root. He received his medical degree from the University of Rochester, did his internship at University Hospitals of Cleveland, and completed his residency at the Cleveland Clinic.

While practicing medicine for a quarter century, his interest in writing never waned. He began honing his craft by attending creative writing workshops and college courses. At first writing solely for himself and his family, he was surprised and gratified when his poems won contests and were published in a variety of literary journals and magazines. He has since published four dozen poems, and been invited to read his work at the George Bush Presidential Library in Texas, the Akron Art Museum in Ohio, and Eckerd College in Florida. His poem, "The People's Republic," was inducted in 2002 into the permanent collection of the George Bush Presidential Library, and reprinted in *Red, White and Blues: Poets on the Promise of America* by the University of Iowa Press.

When not reading or writing, he spends his time swimming, boating, and hiking in Sandusky, Ohio and St. Petersburg, Florida.

BIRD DOG PUBLISHING

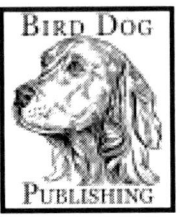

Heart Murmurs: Poems by John Vanek
978-1-933964-27-0   120 pgs. $15

Faces and Voices: Tales by Larry Smith
1-933964-04-9   136 pgs. $14

Second Story Woman: A Memoir of Second Chances
by Carole Calladine
978-1-933964-12-6   226 pgs. $15

256 Zones of Gray: Poems
by Rob Smith
978-1-933964-16-4   80 pgs. $14

Another Life: Collected Poems by Allen Frost
978-1-933964-10-2   176 pgs. $14

Winter Apples: Poems by Paul S. Piper
978-1-933964-08-9   88 pgs. $14

Lake Effect: Poems by Laura Treacy Bentley
1-933964-05-7   108 pgs. $14

Depression Days on an Appalachian Farm: Poems
by Robert L. Tener
1-933964-03-0   80 pgs. $14

120 Charles Street, The Village:
Journals & Other Writings 1949-1950 by Holly Beye
0-933087-99-3   240 pgs. $15

BIRD DOG PUBLISHING
A division of Bottom Dog Press, Inc.
Order Online at: http://smithdocs.net/BirdDogy/BirdDogPage.html

Recent Books by Bottom Dog Press

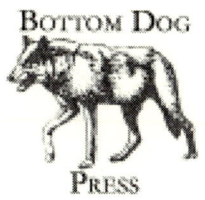

Bar Stories edited by Nan Byrne
978-1-933964-09-6   168 pgs. $14

An Unmistakable Shade of Red & The Obama Chronicles
by Mary E. Weems
978-1-933964-18-8   80 pgs. $15

Cleveland Poetry Scenes: A Panorama and Anthology
eds. Nina Gibans, Mary Weems, Larry Smith
978-1933964-17-1   304 pgs. $20

d.a.levy & the mimeograph revolution
eds. Ingrid Swanberg & Larry Smith
1-933964-07-3 276 pgs. & dvd $25

Our Way of Life: Poems by Ray McNiece
978-1-933964-14-0   128 pgs. $14

Hunger Artist: Childhood in the Suburbs
by Joanne Jacobson
978-1-933964-11-9   132 pgs. $16

Come Together: Imagine Peace
eds. Ann Smith, Larry Smith, Philip Metres
978-1-933964-22-5   224 pgs. $18

Evensong: Contemporary American Poets on Spirituality
eds. Gerry LaFemina & Chad Prevost
ISBN 1-933964-01-4   276 pgs. $18

Bottom Dog Press
Order Online at:
http://smithdocs.net

Printed in the United States
216813BV00001B/3/P